Pocket Guide to
INFLAMMATORY BOWEL DISEASE

Pocket Guide to
INFLAMMATORY BOWEL DISEASE

Edited by

Sunanda V. Kane, MD, MSPH

Assistant Professor of Medicine
University of Chicago
Pritzker School of Medicine
Chicago, Illinois

Marla C. Dubinsky, MD

Assistant Professor of Pediatrics
David Geffen School of Medicine
University of California, Los Angeles
Los Angeles, California

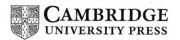
CAMBRIDGE
UNIVERSITY PRESS

CAMBRIDGE UNIVERSITY PRESS
Cambridge, New York, Melbourne, Madrid, Cape Town, Singapore,
São Paulo

Cambridge University Press
40 West 20th Street, New York, NY 10011-4211, USA

www.cambridge.org
Information on this title: www.cambridge.org/9780521672399

First published 2005

Printed in the United States of America

A catalog record for this publication is available from the British Library.

Library of Congress Cataloging in Publication Data

Pocket guide to inflammatory bowel disease / edited by Sunanda V.
Kane, Marla C. Dubinsky.
   p. cm.
Includes bibliographical references and index.
ISBN 0-521-67239-2 (pbk.)
1. Inflammatory bowel disease – Handbooks, manuals, etc.
[DNLM: 1. Inflammatory Bowel Disease – Handbooks. WI 39 P739 2005]
I. Kane, Sunanda.   II. Dubinsky, Marla.   III. Title.
RC862.I53P63   2005
616.3′44 – dc22   2005006201

ISBN-13   978-0-521-67239-9 paperback
ISBN-10   0-521-67239-2 paperback

Contents

Tables

Preface

This handbook is the product of a shared dream of the editors. While there are several fine, comprehensive textbooks available on the subject of inflammatory bowel diseases, we felt there was a need for a different type of book, focused on direct patient care.

The *Pocket Guide to Inflammatory Bowel Disease* is written for busy health care providers on the "front lines." It is meant to be consulted for quick answers on the go, to help anyone who cares for IBD patients identify key problems and make decisions about treatment. The experiences of the editors and contributors as we lectured around the country inspired the format and content of the guidebook – the symptoms that patients complained of most were often the most difficult to triage for the nonspecialist, and the majority of the questions we fielded centered on these issues.

It was our goal to produce a small, easy-to-use guide with practical clinical application covering symptoms, medications, and therapies. Whether on the phone, on the wards, or in the examining room, we hope that this book will be a trusted resource for practitioners caring for patients with IBD.

Sunanda V. Kane
Marla C. Dubinsky

Foreword

Once little known and poorly understood, the inflammatory bowel diseases, ulcerative colitis and Crohn's disease, have undergone a remarkable progression during the past 50 years with new definitive concepts of pathogenesis involving genetic, microbial, and immunological mechanisms, and increased recognition of the varied clinical aspects and complications. Indeed, few diseases in gastroenterology present as diverse an array of clinical problems as the inflammatory bowel diseases. This expansion of scientific knowledge (e.g., epithelial, microbial interactions, cytokines and inflammatory mediators, and neuro-immune interactions) has produced a cascade of publications: textbooks, monographs, reviews, scientific papers, and countless lectures. In addition, characterization of the molecular nature of the IBD inflammatory reaction has identified new therapeutic molecules with differing mechanisms of action and clinical applications, converting the "art" of IBD management to the "science" of IBD therapy.

The wealth of new scientific knowledge of IBD has created the need for a well-organized, authoritative, clinical guide to ulcerative colitis and Crohn's disease outlining the clinical course, complications, and response to therapy; the management of special clinical situations including the pediatric patient and the elderly patient; and the appropriate approaches to diagnosis and management. This need has been admirably met in this excellent publication by Drs. Sunanda Kane and Marla Dubinsky and their talented contributing authors, providing a useful clinical guide to the current practical management of the IBD patient.

This publication is highly recommended to all physicians involved in the study and management of IBD patients, including gastroenterology trainees, nurses, and advanced students who will learn much from this well-organized and authoritative contribution to the IBD literature.

> Joseph B. Kirsner, MD, PhD
> The Louis Block Distinguished
> Service Professor of Medicine
> The University of Chicago

Contributing Authors

Maria T. Abreu, MD
Associate Professor of Medicine
Director of the Inflammatory Bowel
   Disease Center
Mount Sinai Medical Center
New York, NY

Robynne Chutkan, MD
Assistant Professor of Medicine
Georgetown University Hospital
Washington, DC

Marla C. Dubinsky, MD
Director, Pediatric Inflammatory Bowel
   Disease Center
Cedars-Sinai Medical Center
Assistant Professor of Pediatrics
David Geffen School of Medicine
University of California, Los Angeles
Los Angeles, CA

Sonia Friedman, MD
Director of Clinical Research, IBD Center
Associate Physician, Brigham and
  Women's Hospital
Boston, MA

Laura Harrell, MD
Gastroenterology Fellow
Department of Medicine
Section of Gastroenterology
University of Chicago
Chicago, IL

Debra. J. Helper, MD
Associate Professor of Clinical Medicine
Director, Inflammatory Bowel Disease Center
Division of Gastroenterology
Indiana University School of Medicine
Indianapolis, IN

Erin Horowitz, RD, CSP
Clinical Dietitian
Pediatric Inflammatory Bowel Disease Center
Cedars-Sinai Medical Center
Los Angeles, CA

Kim L. Isaacs, MD, PhD
Associate Professor of Medicine
Division of Gastroenterology and Hepatology
University of North Carolina at Chapel Hill
Chapel Hill, NC

Sunanda V. Kane, MD, MSPH
Assistant Professor of Medicine
Section of Gastroenterology
Center for Inflammatory Bowel Diseases
University of Chicago
Pritzker School of Medicine
Chicago, IL

Joshua R. Korzenik, MD
Co-director, MGH Crohn's and Colitis Center
Massachusetts General Hospital
Assistant Professor of Medicine
Harvard Medical School
Boston, MA

Edward V. Loftus, Jr., MD
Associate Professor of Medicine
Mayo Medical School
Consultant, Division of Gastroenterology
   and Hepatology
Mayo Clinic
Rochester, MN

Uma Mahadevan, MD
Associate Director of Clinical Research
Center for Colitis and Crohn's Disease
Assistant Professor of Medicine
Division of Gastroenterology
University of California, San Francisco
San Francisco, CA

Kimberly Persley, MD
Assistant Professor of Medicine
University of Texas Southwestern
Medical School
Presbyterian Hospital of Dallas
Dallas, TX

David T. Rubin, MD
Assistant Professor of Medicine
Director of Clinical Education for
Gastroenterology
Center for Inflammatory Bowel Diseases and
MacLean Center for Clinical Medical Ethics
University of Chicago Pritzker School of Medicine
Chicago, IL

Ellen J. Scherl, MD
Associate Professor of Medicine
Director, Inflammatory Bowel Disease Center
Weill Medical College of Cornell University
New York Presbyterian Hospital – Cornell
New York, NY

Douglas M. Weine, MD
Internal Medicine Resident
Department of Medicine
New York Weill Cornell Medical Center
New York, NY

PART ONE

Basic Overviews

CHAPTER 1

Introduction to Ulcerative Colitis

Ulcerative colitis (UC) is one of the two major groups of chronic idiopathic inflammatory bowel disease (IBD). UC is a worldwide disorder that primarily affects young adults between the ages of 20 and 40 years, but the disease may present at any age. There appears to be a genetic susceptibility that is only partly understood. Certain racial and ethnic groups tend to be more prone to UC than other groups. The familial incidence of ulcerative colitis has been recognized for many years but specific genes have yet to be identified. The cause remains unknown but environmental, immunologic, and psychological factors are thought to be contributors to the etiology and pathogenesis of ulcerative colitis.

CLINICAL FEATURES

The major symptoms of ulcerative colitis include diarrhea, rectal bleeding, and abdominal pain. Disease of moderate or severe activity may be associated with systemic symptoms such as anorexia, nausea, vomiting, fever, and fatigue. Extraintestinal manifestations include arthritis, skin changes, eye changes, or evidence of liver disease. These extracolonic findings are usually related to the activity of the colitis and resolve when the colonic inflammation is controlled. Endoscopically, inflammation begins in the rectum and extends proximally. Approximately 37% of patients will have pancolitis, 17% will have disease extending beyond the sigmoid but not involving the entire colon, 46% will have disease limited to the rectum and rectosigmoid.

COMPLICATIONS

The complications of ulcerative colitis may be classified as *local* or *systemic*. Local complications include the development of fissures, abscesses, or hemorrhoids. Local complications are a direct reflection of mucosal inflammation and its extension. Severe complications include massive hemorrhage, perforation, toxic megacolon, strictures, pseudopolyps, and colon cancer. Systemic complications include the extra-colonic manifestations, but also weight loss and anemia.

THERAPY

The initial treatment of ulcerative colitis is usually medical. Surgery is reserved for specific complications and intractability of disease activity. Assessment of disease extent and severity is important in effective management. Limited, mild disease can usually be treated on an outpatient basis. More severe disease may need treatment in the hospital setting. The goal of medical therapy is to control intestinal inflammation. The principal drugs used in the therapy of ulcerative colitis are the salicylates (sulfasalazine and mesalamine), corticosteroids, and immunosuppressives (azathioprine, 6-mercaptopurine, and cyclosporine). Once the disease is in remission, patients are usually maintained with 5-ASAs or purine metabolites (AZA and 6-MP). Approximately 20%–25% of patients will require colectomy during the course of the disease. Indications for colectomy include: severe attacks failing to respond to medical therapy, complications of a severe attack, chronic continuous disease with impaired quality of life, dysplasia, or carcinoma.

PROGNOSIS

Most patients with ulcerative colitis have intermittent attacks of their disease. A few patients will have only a single attack. Approximately 10%–15% of patients will have a chronic continuous course. Patients with extensive or pancolitis are much more likely to have severe attacks than those patients with limited disease. Finally, colectomy rate is higher in patients with more extensive disease.

CHAPTER 2

Introduction to Crohn's Disease

Crohn's disease is a form of inflammatory bowel disease that can manifest with a variety of clinical features. It is a chronic inflammatory disease involving the gastrointestinal tract and is characterized by episodes of acute flares of symptoms and periods of remission. Crohn's disease may be diagnosed at any age but is commonly diagnosed in young adults. It is more common in industrialized nations in northern climates with the highest prevalence of Crohn's disease found in northern Europe, the United Kingdom, and North America. The prevalence of Crohn's disease in the United States ranges from 26 to 199 cases per 100,000 persons. It affects all ethnic groups but is more common in white populations and carries a slightly greater risk in the Jewish population, especially in Jews of European descent. The incidence of Crohn's disease in African Americans is also rising in recent years. The cause of Crohn's disease is not entirely understood but is likely the result of an individual's genetic makeup and environmental exposures.

CLINICAL FEATURES

Crohn's disease may involve any portion of the gastrointestinal tract from the mouth to the anus. The inflammation in Crohn's disease is typically discontinuous with areas of normal mucosa in-between areas of inflamed mucosa. The inflammation may involve the full thickness of the bowel wall, which can lead to the development of large and deep ulcerations. Many complications can potentially result from the inflammatory process found in Crohn's disease. Chronic inflammation can lead to stricturing of the bowel lumen, sometimes resulting in bowel obstruction. Abscesses or fistulas (connections between the intestines and another loop of bowel, the bladder, vagina, or skin) may also develop.

Symptoms of Crohn's disease vary depending on the location of disease involvement and the extent and severity of inflammation. Crohn's disease is often categorized by disease location and disease behavior. Disease behavior can be described as predominantly inflammatory, fibrostenoic, or penetrating in nature. Patients may experience abdominal pain, diarrhea, fever, weight loss, or fatigue. Some patients develop perirectal abscesses or fistula to the skin surrounding the anus. Patients may also experience extraintestinal manifestations such as arthritis, skin rashes including *pyoderma gangrenosum* or *erythema nodosum*, inflammation of the eye, or diseases involving the liver.

THERAPY

Treatment of Crohn's disease depends on disease location and the severity of disease. There are two stages of therapy in the treatment of inflammatory bowel disease, the induction of remission and the maintenance of remission. Aminosalicylate preparations are sometimes used for treatment of active disease and maintenance of remission. Antibiotics are also used to treat active disease. Corticosteroids are sometimes needed on a short-term basis to induce remission. Newer corticosteroids with fewer systemic side effects are now available and widely used to treat active disease. Many patients require treatment with immunomodulators such as azathioprine or 6-mercaptopurine. These medications are used as maintenance drugs and are useful in patients who have mild-to-moderate disease or steroid-dependent disease.

In recent years, there has been substantial development in biologic therapies for the treatment of Crohn's disease. The most widely used biologic therapy is infliximab, a chimeric monoclonal antibody against a proinflammatory cytokine, TNFα. The development and success of infliximab has revolutionized the treatment of moderate-to-severe disease. Surgery remains an important therapeutic option when medical therapy has failed.

PROGNOSIS

Crohn's disease is a lifelong disease, but with proper diagnosis and management of the disease and its complications, patients often lead healthy and normal lives.

PART TWO

Patient Symptoms

CHAPTER 3

Abdominal Pain

I. CONDITIONS TO CONSIDER

▤ In Crohn's disease
- Acute obstruction
- Perforation
- Abscess
- Active inflammatory disease

▤ In ulcerative colitis
- Perforation
- Toxic megacolon

▤ In either diagnosis
- Peptic ulcer disease
- Pancreatitis
- Gallstones, kidney stones
- Acute appendicitis
- Medication-related pain

- Irritable bowel syndrome
- Diverticulitis

II. QUESTIONS TO ASK

1. Where is the pain?
- Location can help determine the etiology.

2. What is the character of the pain? Is it crampy, colicky, diffuse, sharp, and so forth?

3. How long has the pain been present?
- A pain present for a few days rules out acute, emergent situations.

4. Is it related to oral intake?

5. Is there anything that relieves the pain?
- Relief with defecation suggests a functional problem, eating suggests peptic ulcer.

6. Are there any other associated symptoms?
- Fevers, diarrhea, bleeding all suggest an inflammatory etiology.

III. TESTS TO ORDER

The physical exam is important, unless the history clearly points to a source.

▥ Blood tests
- CBC to rule out infection
- Chemistry panel for metabolic derangements

- Amylase and lipase for pancreatitis
- C-reactive protein to rule out active inflammatory disease.

■ **X-rays**

- Flat plate to rule out free air, dilated small bowel or colon, stones, stool in right colon
- Ultrasound
- RUQ for cholelithiasis, bilary dilation, pancreas and liver abnormalities
- CT scan to rule out abscess, transmural inflammation, pancreatobiliary sources, appendicitis, vascular abnormalities
- Endoscopy is rarely helpful unless there are other signs or symptoms of inflammation – that is, bleeding, diarrhea.

CHAPTER 4

Arthralgias (Joint Pains)

Joint pains in the IBD patient can be due to a variety of conditions, and treatment depends upon the underlying etiology. Arthralgias can be difficult to treat because they can be related not only to active inflammation, but also can represent common osteoarthritis or a side effect of medications.

I. CONDITIONS TO CONSIDER

- Active IBD
- Osteoarthritis
- Tendonitis
- Secondary inflammatory arthritis
- Fracture

II. QUESTIONS TO ASK

1. Are the joints red, warm, or otherwise "inflamed"?

- This could signal true inflammation versus simple arthralgia that typically accompanies active IBD.

2. How many joints are involved?

- One specific joint could represent either infection or trauma. Multiple joints suggest either drug reaction or active IBD.

3. Was there a recent infusion of infliximab?

- The joint complaints tend to be migratory, polyarticular, and associated with a migratory rash. Patients will usually respond to a Medrol Dosepak or 2 weeks of low-dose prednisone 5–10 mg a day.

4. Is it back pain specifically?

- This could signal another inflammatory condition, ankylosing spondylitis, or possible abscess in patients with Crohn's disease.
- Also you have to consider fracture, spinal stenosis, or even kidney stones.

5. Is it hip pain specifically?

- Fracture or avascular necrosis (the patient on steroids must be warned of the risk of avascular necrosis and osteoporosis).

III. TESTS TO ORDER

- X-rays. Plain films to rule out skeletal abnormalities.
- Consider CT scan for abscess; MRI for other joint and soft tissue conditions.
- ESR and/or CRP to rule out active inflammation.
- ANA, dsDNA, histone antibody, and HLA-B27 to assess for autoimmune arthritis.
- Consider Lyme and parvovirus titers if patient has any travel history.
- Vitamin $D_{1.25}$, vitamin D_{25}, parathyroid hormone, and DEXA scan if patient has risk factors for osteoporosis.
- Consider also a celiac panel.
- Stool: Consider culture for *Yersinia*.

CHAPTER 5

Diarrhea

Diarrhea is one of the common symptoms that indicate a flare of disease activity in inflammatory bowel disease. There are other potential etiologies of diarrhea that run the spectrum from medication side effect to superimposed infection.

I. CONDITIONS TO CONSIDER

- Active IBD
- *C. difficile* infection
- Medication side effect
- Small bowel bacterial overgrowth
- Bile acid diarrhea
- Infectious gastroenteritis
- Lactose intolerance
- Hyperthyroidism

II. QUESTIONS TO ASK

1. What is the nature of the diarrhea?

- Small volume, bloody with tenesmus suggests active rectal inflammation.
- Large volume, nonbloody seen in small intestinal disease such as recurrent CD or infectious enteritis.
- Blood mixed in with diarrhea suggests an active colitic process.
- Does it stop with fasting? In diarrhea caused by malabsorption, stool volume will decrease.

2. How does this compare to baseline stool frequency, consistency, and volume? How did the diarrhea start?

- Many patients with IBD will have altered baseline bowel habits due to disease activity, prior surgeries, and medical therapy.
- Increased diarrhea associated with a flare in disease activity is typically more insidious in onset.
- Acute onset of diarrhea in an otherwise stable baseline is suggestive of an infectious process.

3. What is the patient's current medication history?

- Of the IBD medications commonly used, 5-aminosalicylates may be associated with worsening diarrhea. Osalazine may cause a secretory diarrhea in up to 20% of patients with initiation of therapy.

- Check to see if the patient has recently changed IBD medications. Patients on chronic immuno-suppression such as those on 6-MP, AZA, and maintenance Remicade infusions are at risk for opportunistic infections that may cause diarrhea such as CMV infection.

- NSAIDs may be associated with IBD flares and in addition may cause diarrhea independently as a side effect.

- Recent antibiotic use? If yes, this raises the question of *C. difficile* infection. Note that this can also occur in the absence of antibiotic exposure.

4. Has the patient had any surgery?

- Resection of the terminal ileum may lead to bile acid malabsorption and a subsequent secretory diarrhea related to the bile acids.

- If patients have had > 100 cm of small bowel resected they are at risk for fat and nutrient malabsorption due to decreased surface area of the bowel.

5. Has the patient ever had a bowel stricture? Stricturing disease may lead to small bowel bacterial overgrowth.

6. Is there an association with any type of food intake?

- Acquired carbohydrate malabsorption may occur with disruption of the brush border enzymes during active inflammation.
- Sprue can coexist with Crohn's disease and symptoms may be exacerbated by gluten-containing products.
- Lactose intolerance may coexist with inflammatory bowel disease.
- Certain sugar substitutes such as sorbitol may produce an osmotic diarrhea.

7. Is the diarrhea associated with the menstrual cycle?

Hormonal changes during different points of the menstrual cycle may be associated with increased bowel activity and diarrhea.

III. TESTS TO ORDER

If the diarrhea is mild, supportive therapy can be used but, if persistent, evaluation will likely be required. Evaluation can in part be tailored to the suspected cause or consequence of the diarrhea.

- CBC. In acute inflammation or active inflammatory disease, there may be an elevated white blood cell count and platelet count and anemia.

- Electrolytes. Profuse watery diarrhea may lead to dehydration and potassium depletion, which will need replacement.
- TFTs, B_{12} level, celiac sprue serology are tests that may be performed in certain patients to help delineate the diarrheal process.
- Stool studies. Check for *C. difficile* toxin, bacterial screen, and parasites. *Giardia* may be superimposed on underlying inflammatory bowel disease.
- Stool WBCs. If absent, would argue against an acute infectious colitis. If the stool is very liquid, stool electrolytes can be measured to delineate a secretory from a malabsorptive diarrheal process. Na and K are measured in the stool. A spot fecal fat check can be done to look grossly for fat malabsorption
- Physical exam. Look for signs of dehydration with dry mucus membranes, decreased axillary sweat, and poor skin turgor.
  - On abdominal exam, tenderness suggests active inflammation.
  - Tenderness would be less likely with a bile acid diarrhea or a diarrhea secondary to bacterial overgrowth or lactose intolerance.
- Flexible sigmoidoscopy. Active inflammation as well as pseudomembranes can be identified visually. Biopsies should be performed

to R/O superimposed CMV colitis. This is especially important in patients who are on chronic immunosuppression.

- Breath hydrogen test for bacterial overgrowth and lactose intolerance.

CHAPTER 6

Fatigue

Fatigue is often the most troublesome symptom of IBD. It greatly limits work and social activities and often prevents patients from completing even basic daily routines. It is a major cause of depression in IBD patients. Fatigue stems from a variety of causes and treating each in turn can often make a big difference in a patient's quality of life.

I. CONDITIONS TO CONSIDER

- Active IBD
- Iron-deficiency anemia
- B_{12}/folate deficiency
- Malnutrition
- Electrolyte abnormalities
- Chronic pain
- Depression

- Undiagnosed malignancy
- Drug reaction
- Adrenal insufficiency
- Unrelated viral infection
- TPN line infection
- Pregnancy
- IBD-related arthritis
- Hypothyroidism

II. QUESTIONS TO ASK

1. How long has the fatigue been going on?

- Several days to a week. May be due to increased disease activity, drug reaction, electrolyte abnormality, or line infection.
- Several weeks to months. Worry about something more chronic such as iron/B_{12}/folate deficiency, malnutrition, pregnancy, adrenal insufficiency, IBD-related arthritis, hypothyroidism.
- Several months to years. Harder to correct, but must be investigated. Consider chronic pain, depression, and malignancy.

2. How severe is the fatigue?

- Mild. Usually due to mild lab abnormality, anemia, mild flare, unrelated viral infection.
- Moderate. Can be due to IBD flare, malnutrition, hypothyroidism, or adrenal insufficiency.

- Severe. Must be immediately dealt with because it could indicate a life-threatening condition such as a malignancy, severe anemia, or sepsis.

3. What are some of the associated symptoms?

- Abdominal pain/diarrhea can indicate an IBD flare.
- Weight loss can signal malnutrition, vitamin and mineral deficiencies, or a malignancy.
- Bleeding can cause anemia.
- Chronic pain, depression, inability to leave house. Need a consult with a pain specialist and/or a psychiatrist.
- Dizziness/fainting/arthralgias can indicate adrenal insufficiency or can occur while prednisone is being tapered.
- Fevers/arthritis/arthralgias. Serum sickness-like reaction to infliximab or autoimmune reaction to infliximab.
- Nausea/vomiting could indicate pregnancy (get a urine or serum HCG) or an IBD flare.

4. What else is going on in the patient's life?

- Increased physical or work activity. Can easily cause fatigue in an already chronically ill individual.
- Self-induced vomiting or limiting food intake due to an eating disorder. This is more

common than you might think and contributes to malnutrition in certain IBD patients.

- Nonadherence to medication such as iron, B_{12}, folate, or nutritional supplements. This contributes to anemia and malnutrition.
- Nonadherence to IBD medications resulting in IBD flares.
- OTC medications and certain herbal preparations can cause fatigue. Always examine carefully what the patient is taking. Patients should bring in pill bottles and all OTC medications to the office visit.
- Menstrual cycles that cause some women to feel more fatigued around their periods and also to flare during menstruation.

5. What is the patient's current IBD therapy regimen?

- 6-MP/AZA can cause fatigue as a side effect.
- Infliximab can cause fatigue through several mechanisms: Patients can develop an autoimmune reaction consisting of DNA. With long lapses between infusions, patients can also develop a serum sickness-like reaction consisting of fevers, arthralgias, and fatigue.
- Prednisone. After taking prednisone for as few as 3 months, patients can develop adrenal insufficiency after the prednisone is tapered. Patients tapered to 10 mg or less should be

tested by either an A. M. cortisol level or a cortisol stimulation test. In addition, the process of tapering prednisone itself can cause fatigue and arthralgias.

III. TESTS TO ORDER

With fatigue that lasts more than a week, the patient should come in and be evaluated.

- CBC, B_{12}, folate, electrolyte levels, albumin, TSH. Will assess for anemia, infection, malnutrition, hypothyroidism, and electrolyte imbalances
- A. M. cortisol level, cortisol stimulation tests in appropriate patients
- Calorie counts. Consult with nutritionist in appropriate patients
- Blood, urine, and stool cultures. In febrile patients or in immunosuppressed patients who are moderately to severely fatigued to rule out an occult infection
- Urine or serum HCG. In women of childbearing age
- ANA and anti-dsDNA. For patients on infliximab
- Psychiatric evaluation. For patients with depression or eating disorders
- Pain specialist evaluation. For patients with chronic pain

- Physical exam. Look for tachycardia, hypotension, lymphadenopathy, thyromegaly, abdominal mass, blood on rectal exam
- Back and spine x-rays. For certain patients with joint complaints.

CHAPTER 7

Fever

Fever in IBD can signal disease activity, an IBD complication, or a drug reaction. It can range from a low-grade fever responsive to Tylenol to high fevers and shaking chills that require hospitalization. Fever in IBD has a long list of causes and only careful questioning and examination will elucidate the problem.

I. CONDITIONS TO CONSIDER

- Active IBD
- Intra-abdominal perforation
- Intra-abdominal abscess
- Drug reaction
- Postoperative fever
- TPN-line infection
- Unrelated viral or bacterial infection
- Infection due to immunosuppression

- Deep vein thrombosis
- Kidney stone
- A medical condition that may be related to IBD (cholecystitis/cholangitis/pancreatitis)
- A medical condition that is not necessarily related to IBD (appendicitis, diverticulitis, myocardial infarction, CVA, hematologic malignancy)

II. QUESTIONS TO ASK

1. How high is the fever?
- Low-grade fever. May be postoperative, increased IBD activity, or drug reaction. Will abate when the precipitant is treated or removed.
- High-grade fever. May be something more serious such as a bowel perforation or an abscess. Usually requires at least an ER visit.

2. How long has the fever lasted?
- A day or two. Can be increased IBD activity or any other condition that has just started. Will require removal of precipitant and/or correlation with other symptoms.
- Longer than a couple of days. Needs evaluation and further testing.

3. What other symptoms are associated with the fever?
- Abdominal pain. Worry about abscess, perforation.

- Diarrhea. Worry about increased IBD activity.
- Back pain. Worry about kidney stone.
- Right upper quadrant/epigastric pain. Worry about biliary/pancreatic complication.
- Chest pain. Worry about MI, PE, bronchitis, and pneumonia.
- Upper respiratory symptoms. Worry about common cold, sinusitis.
- Post-op fever. If persistent, needs thorough evaluation.
- Asymmetric leg swelling. Worry about DVT.
- Abnormal blood count. Worry about infection or malignancy.

4. What else is the patient doing?

- Increased physical activity resulting in dehydration. When combined with diarrhea, physical activity can cause dehydration and thus a fever.
- NSAID use. Can trigger bowel activity and thus cause a fever.
- Antibiotic use. Can trigger bowel activity and thus cause a fever.
- OTC preparation use. May rarely cause a fever due to a drug reaction.
- In ulcerative colitis, patients can flare when they stop smoking; in Crohn's disease, cigarettes can increase severity of illness.

5. What is the patient's current IBD therapy regimen?

- Sulfasalazine. Can cause a drug-induced fever in up to 25%–30% of patients. This is due to the sulfapyridine component of the drug.
- 6-MP/AZA. Can cause a drug-induced fever in up to 5% of patients. This usually occurs within the first month of therapy and is reversible when the drug is stopped.
- 6-MP/AZA + 5-ASA agents. Rarely can cause a febrile neutropenia in combination.
- 6-MP/AZA + allopurinol. Can cause a profound leukopenia in combination and can present as a fever.
- Infliximab. Fevers can be associated with an infusion reaction or can be due to infection. Fevers can also be associated with a serum sickness-like reaction due to long periods between infliximab doses.
- TPN. Worry about line infection and have blood and line cultures done immediately.

III. TESTS TO ORDER

Often, patients will need a thorough evaluation. Depending upon the patient's symptoms, the following tests should be performed:

- CBC with differential. Will help diagnose infection, leukopenia, malignancy, and anemia

- Electrolytes. Will assess for dehydration
- Urinalysis. For infection or blood indicating a kidney stone
- Stool studies. Always check bacterial cultures, *C. difficile* toxin, *Giardia* antigen if the patient has increased gas and bloating and has done some outdoor travel, and ova and parasites if the patient is on immunosuppressives
- Blood and line cultures if the patient has a central line. Will rule out sepsis
- Physical exam. Take the patient's temperature. Look for CVA or abdominal tenderness. Listen for pneumonia. Check for tachycardia, hypotension. Look for asymmetric leg swelling
- CT scan of the abdomen/pelvis. Will rule out a perforation/abscess/kidney stone/biliary or pancreatic complication

CHAPTER 8

Nausea

Within the context of inflammatory bowel disease, nausea can be due to any of a number of causes seen in people without IBD or it may be due to a recurrence of the disease, a complication of the disease, or a side effect of therapy.

I. CONDITIONS TO CONSIDER

- Gastroesophageal reflux disease
- Obstruction (small bowel or gastric outlet) due to stricture or adhesions
- Active IBD, especially Crohn's disease of the upper GI tract
- Medication side effect
- Adrenal insufficiency (in patients previously on chronic corticosteroid therapy)

- Liver disease (hepatitis related to medication, infection, or malignancy)
- Gallbladder disease
- Central causes

II. QUESTIONS TO ASK

1. Is the nausea persistent or only during part of the day?
- Morning nausea could be related to medications, but do not forget about the possibility of pregnancy. Many women with IBD may have irregular menstrual periods, and may not know that they are pregnant.

2. How long has the patient been nauseated?
- A day suggests something acute, as opposed to days to weeks, which could signal worsening disease or medication reaction.

3. Is the patient also vomiting?
- Vomiting along with nausea may suggest obstruction and should focus your attention on more acute conditions.

4. What is the nature of the emesis?
- Old food would suggest gastric outlet obstruction.
- Blood would suggest ulcer disease, bleeding from a complication such as primary sclerosing

cholangitis with variceal bleeding, or proximal
small bowel active Crohn's disease.

5. Is it related to food?

- Nausea that is improved with food may signal
  peptic ulcer disease.
- Nausea that is not relieved with food intake,
  or made worse, may be disease- or medication-
  related.

6. Is there associated abdominal pain?

- Crampy abdominal pain would suggest active
  small bowel disease.
- Sharp pain radiating through to the back could
  be pancreatitis.
- Colicky right upper quadrant pain would be
  more consistent with a biliary source.
- Burning epigastric pain might be caused by
  ulcer or gastroesophageal reflux.
- Severe colicky abdominal pain would suggest
  obstruction.

7. Is the patient's abdomen distended or swollen?

- Significant abdominal distension would be wor-
  risome for distal obstruction.
- Proximal small bowel or gastric outlet obstruction may occur without significant distension
  but can cause a great deal of nausea.
- Severe colicky pain with distension and vomiting would suggest high-grade obstruction and
  requires immediate evaluation.

8. What medications and supplements is the patient currently taking?

- Many IBD therapies are notorious for nausea as a side effect. They include (but are not limited to) metronidazole, azathioprine/6-mercaptopurine (with or without pancreatitis or hepatitis), sulfasalazine, methotrexate, narcotics (either central nausea or due to decreased intestinal motility).
- Nausea/vomiting is usually an isolated symptom and may be temporally related to the ingestion of the medication.

9. What actions and/or medications could the patient take for immediate relief?

- If symptoms are mild, consider trial of proton pump inhibitor.
- Metoclopramide may be useful if dysmotility is suspected but is contraindicated if there is a possibility of obstruction.
- If symptoms are temporally associated with administration of a medication, adjust or hold it to see if the nausea abates. In the case of metronidazole, an acceptable alternative might be used, or a trial of the enteric-coated (375 mg) pill can be employed.
- Similarly, with sulfasalazine, the Entab formulation may be better tolerated. Alternative mesalamine products could be substituted at

equivalent doses because they lack the sulfapyridine moiety present in sulfasalazine and
are less likely to cause nausea.
- Narcotic use should be minimized.

III. TESTS TO ORDER

When patients are unable to keep down any fluids, have them go to the ER and be evaluated for
physical findings of obstruction; supplement with
a plain film of the abdomen/obstructive series.

- Abdominal CT scan. If suspicion is strong but
  there is no clear evidence of obstruction on
  the plain films, consider this to evaluate for
  obstruction by fluid-filled loops of bowel, or a
  closed-loop obstruction due to adhesion
- RUQ ultrasound would help document any
  cholecystitis
- Blood tests looking at:
  - amylase and lipase, other liver enzymes
  - CBC
  - inflammatory markers such as CRP
  - sedimentation rate
  - fasting morning cortisol (as indicated)
  - Cortrosyn stimulation test (as indicated if
    adrenal insufficiency is suspected)
  - electrolytes including magnesium and cal-
    cium (derangements may cause dysmotility

and exacerbate nausea in patients with vomiting and/or diarrhea)

- UGI endoscopy. Evaluates active upper GI tract Crohn's disease, peptic ulcer disease, gastric outlet, or proximal small bowel obstruction that may be relieved by endoscopic dilation and/or steroid injection
- Enteroclysis or video capsule endoscopy (VCE). Further testing of the small bowel may need to be performed to clearly demonstrate active small bowel disease as the source of nausea. VCE is contraindicated in patients suspected of having obstruction and should only be performed in patients with IBD after radiographic small bowel imaging reveals no evidence of narrowing
- MRI of brain and brainstem if the central source is considered a possibility

CHAPTER 9

Rash

Certain skin conditions can herald the onset of active disease, some can run an independent course from any gastrointestinal symptoms.

I. CONDITIONS TO CONSIDER

- Infectious conditions
- *Erythema nodosum*
- *Pyoderma gangrenosum*
- Cutaneous Crohn's disease
- Psoriasis/eczema
- Skin cancer

II. QUESTIONS TO ASK

1. **How active are the patient's gastrointestinal symptoms?** *Erythema nodosum* and cutaneous Crohn's, as well as psoriasis or eczema are more

likely to be active when gastrointestinal symptoms
are active.

2. What does the rash look like?

- A diffuse red rash suggests drug reaction or
  allergies.
- A "band" of erythema suggests herpes. Nodules
  on the extremities could be *E. nodosum, P. gangrenosum,* or cutaneous Crohn's.

3. Has the patient started any new medications?

**4. Does the patient have risk factors for skin
cancer?**

5. Has the patient been on steroids?

- Acne can be a side effect of steroid therapy.
- Steroids predispose patients to infectious
  agents and poor wound healing.

III. TESTS TO ORDER

- Examination of the rash is important because a
  biopsy may be necessary
- In most instances, a history is more important
  than any tests, and a referral to a dermatologist
  when a punch biopsy is needed is prudent

CHAPTER 10

Rectal Bleeding

Rectal bleeding is one of the key symptoms that signal possible disease activity. However, bleeding as an individual symptom runs a full spectrum from simple hemorrhoids to life-threatening hemorrhage. It is the careful consideration of the accompanying symptoms that helps appropriately triage the patient.

I. CONDITIONS TO CONSIDER

- Active IBD
- Fistula bleeding
- Hemorrhoids/fissure
- Gynecologic bleeding
- Concurrent colitis

II. QUESTIONS TO ASK

1. What is the nature of the bleeding?

- Drops on the toilet paper. Suggests hemorrhoids or other anal canal abnormalities.
- Mixed in with stool. Suggests possible active colitis or ileitis.
- Clots. May signal active bleeding.
- Spontaneous bleeding. Blood seen with or without bowel movements may signal very active disease.

2. How long has the bleeding been going on?

- Patients may wait for a significant amount of time before calling the office. The longer the patient has been bleeding, the more time it will take to resolve.

3. What are some of the associated symptoms?

- Rectal pain. This can be associated with Crohn's disease, ulcerative colitis, or an anal fissure.
- Urgency. This signals inflammation in the rectum.
- Straining. Very active left-sided disease may cause a relative constipation on the right side of the colon that results in straining. This also can be associated with rectal inflammation.
- Diarrhea. This may signal active disease or another concurrent colitis.

4. What is the patient's current medication history?

- NSAID use. Estimates suggest that regular NSAID use is associated with a 30% risk of precipitating a flare of symptoms.
- Antibiotic use. Certain antibiotics, particularly the penicillin-based ones, can cause gastrointestinal symptoms as well as *C. difficile* infection.
- In ulcerative colitis patients, smoking cessation can precipitate a flare, in Crohn's disease continued smoking can potentiate disease activity.
- Menstrual cycle. Women may notice a pattern of more active symptoms related to their menstrual cycle, and symptoms can be treated rather than a true flare of IBD.

5. What is the patient's current IBD therapy?

- Prescription medicines
  - Patients who stopped taking their maintenance medications are likely to flare.
  - Patients may be taking a fraction of what you may think they are taking.
  - Other patients may have recently been started on a 5-ASA compound.
  - Hypersensitivity, that is, worse bleeding, can occur in up to 7% of patients prescribed this class of medicines.

- Ask women about changes in their oral contraceptive preparations; any change may lead to a disease flare.
- OTC preparations.
  - Patients will not admit to supplements or OTC therapies.
  - NSAIDs, compounds containing magnesium, may cause diarrhea and precipitate a flare.
- CAM. Many herbal compounds have unknown toxicities and must be considered in the differential.

III. TESTS TO ORDER

If you decide to have the patient come in to be evaluated, here are some considerations:

- CBC. Do you have a baseline? This will help tell the chronicity and/or severity of the bleeding
- Stool studies. Do not waste your time with fecal leukocytes because they will be present if there is visible blood. Remember to check for *C. difficile* toxin along with appropriate bacterial cultures depending on the patient's history for potential exposure. Patients do not necessarily need a history of antibiotic use to have a *C. difficile* colitis

- Physical exam. Check for pallor, tachycardia, skin turgor, and overall appearance. A rectal exam is imperative
- Flexible sigmoidoscopy. Not just an endoscopic interpretation; make sure you get biopsies if there is active disease to rule out CMV colitis

CHAPTER 11

The Red Eye

Certain eye conditions can be associated with IBD, and should be taken seriously when a patient calls with this particular complaint.

I. CONDITIONS TO CONSIDER

- Episcleritis
- Uveitis
- Corneal abrasion or injury
- Infectious conjunctivitis
- Allergic reaction

II. QUESTIONS TO ASK

1. Is there vision loss?
- This is an ophthalmologic emergency and the patient should be seen immediately.

2. Does the eye hurt?

- This could also signal a progressive condition and the patient should be seen by an ophthalmologist, not just an optometrist.

3. Has the patient been on steroids?

- Cataracts, infections, and retinal detachment are all complications of steroid use.

III. TESTS TO ORDER

The patient should be seen quickly.

- If there is eye pain or vision loss, the patient should be seen within hours
- Slit-lamp examination. Even without pain or loss of vision, the patient should probably be referred to an ophthalmologist who will consider this or other tests.

PART THREE

Medications and Other Therapies

CHAPTER 12

Medications Used in IBD

Every patient with IBD has to be treated as an individual; there is no "cookbook" management with these conditions. Disease location, disease severity, patient preferences, and physician experience all play a role in deciding which medication or combination of medicines is appropriate. Table 12.1, Commonly prescribed medications for treating IBD, lists medications that are available by prescription and used to treat IBD. This list is not exhaustive but, as we continue to develop more targeted and specific therapies, it will change. Off-label therapies are certainly available, but are too new to be discussed here.

Table 12.1. **Commonly prescribed medications for treating IBD**

Drug	Class	FDA IBD Indication	Common Uses
Prednisone	Systemic corticosteroid	None	Mod–severe UC, CD
Budesonide (Entocort)	Local-acting corticosteroid	Mild–mod ileocecal CD	Ileocecal CD
Cortfoam, Cortenema	Topical/Rectal Steroid	None	Proctitis; active left-sided symptoms
pH-controlled mesalamine (Asacol)	5-ASA	Mild–mod UC	Colitis
Time-released mesalamine (Pentasa)	5-ASA	Mild–mod UC	Small and large bowel CD, UC
Balsalazide (Colazal)	5-ASA	Mild–mod UC	Colitis
Olsalazine (Dipentum)	5-ASA	Maintenance of UC	UC
Sulfasalazine (Azulfidine)	5-ASA	None	Colitis
Canasa	Topical 5–ASA	None	Proctitis

Dosing	Common AE	Special Considerations
1–2 mg/kg to max of 40–60 mg	Cushingoid features: weight gain, acne, mood changes	Not for long-term use; pt well on steroids is not in true remission. May affect growth in children
9 mg po for 6 wk, 6 mg for 2 wk, then off	Same as prednisone, but occurs less frequently	Safer than prednisone, but not for long-term use. Used also for collagenous colitis, microscopic colitis
Rectal application qd-bid	Weight gain, headache	Some systemic absorption
2.4–4.8 g po (400 mg tablets)	Headache, diarrhea, abdominal pain	3–7% hypersensitivity; nephritis is idiosyncratic
2–4 g po (250 mg capsules)	Headache, diarrhea, abdominal pain	3–7% hypersensitivity; nephritis is idiosyncratic
6.75 g po (750 mg capsules)	Headache, diarrhea, abdominal pain	3–7% hypersensitivity, nephritis is idiosyncratic
2–3 g po (500 mg capsules)	Diarrhea	Only indicated for maintenance
3–6 g po (500 mg capsules)	Rash, n/v, headache	Dose response limited by AE; enteric-coated tablets may improve tolerance; folic acid supplementation recommended
500 mg pr qd-bid (500 mg suppository)	Bloating, gas	Can be used in combination with po 5-ASA

(*continued*)

Table 12.1 (*continued*)

Drug	Class	FDA IBD Indication	Common Uses
Rowasa enema	Topical 5-ASA	None	Proctitis; left-sided colitis
Azathioprine (Azasan, Imuran)	Immunomodulator	None	More commonly CD, but also UC
6-MP (Purinethol)	Immunomodulator	None	Commonly CD, but also UC
Cyclosporine (Neoral, Sandimmune)	Immunomodulator	None	Severe UC and CD, fistulizing CD
Methotrexate	Immunomodulator	None	CD
Tacrolimus (Protopic)	Topical ointment	None	Cutaneous, perineal, perianal CD, *P. gangrenosum*
Tacrolimus (Prograf)	Immunomodulator	None	Severe UC and CD; fistulizing CD
Thalidomide	Immunomodulator	Orphan use for CD	Mod–severe CD

Dosing	Common AE	Special Considerations
4 g pr qhs (4 g enema)	Bloating, gas, incontinence	Often used in combination with po 5-ASA
2–2.5 mg/kg body weight po (50, 75, 100 mg tablets)	Neutropenia, pancreatitis, rash, fevers	TPMT testing suggested prior to initiation
1–1.5 mg/kg body weight po (50 mg tablets)	Neutropenia, pancreatitis, rash, fevers	TPMT testing suggested prior to initiation
2–4 mg/kg IV, then $2 \times$ IV dose po	Seizures, HTN, nephrotoxicity, hypomagnesemia	Levels need to be monitored to avoid AE; Bactrim for prophylaxis of PCP
25 mg SQ/IMr 12 wk, then 15 mg SQ maintenance	Mucositis, hepatotoxicity, pulmonary fibrosis	Pregnancy, category X; folic acid supplementation recommended
Strength 0.03–0.1%; apply to affected area qd-bid	Itching, burning of skin	Minimal absorption, but levels should be monitored initially
0.1–0.3 mg/kg/dose po bid	N/V, heartburn, diarrhea, nephrotoxicity	Levels must be monitored, risks may outweigh potential benefits;, available in cream
50–250 mg po qd	Neuropathy, sedation	Pregnancy, category X

(*continued*)

Table 12.1 (*continued*)

Drug	Class	FDA IBD Indication	Common Uses
Ciprofloxacin	Antibiotic	None	Fistulizing and colonic CD
Metronidazole (Flagyl)	Antibiotic	None	Fistulizing and colonic CD
Infliximab (Remicade)	Biologic agent	Inflammatory and fistulizing CD, active and maintenance	CD, UC, pouchitis, EIM of IBD

Dosing	Common AE	Special Considerations
500 mg – 1g po qd	Rash, headache, diarrhea	Interacts with nutritional supplements
500–1000 mg po qd	Potential interaction with alcohol, metallic taste, neuropathy	Long-term use often limited by neuropathy, dose reduction may decrease risk
5–10 mg/kg IV 0,2,6 wk induction, then q 8 wk	Infusion reactions, delayed hypersensitivity, URI symptoms, other infections	PPD must be performed prior to initiating due to increased risk of TB; possible to develop either intolerance or nonresponse over time

CHAPTER 13

Infliximab and Its Management

Prior to your patients' first infusions of infliximab, perform PPD to rule out latent TB. If anergic, consider an entire anergy panel or chest x-ray to document lack of evidence for TB.

I. CONDITIONS TO CONSIDER

- Immunomodulator history. Are patients on one? Should they be on one? Did patients have adverse reactions to them in the past?
  - During infusion, assess patient's reactions, vital signs, and whether there is rash, wheezing, or swelling to indicate an impending serious problem. If so, shut off the infusion.
  - If mild reactions, give diphenhydramine 50 mg IV along with acetaminophen 650 mg po and consider steroids.

- If patient rigoring, meperidine 25 mg–50 mg SQ/IV will help, although patient is going to have to be accompanied home if narcotics are given.

II. QUESTIONS TO ASK

1. Does patient need to continue infliximab therapy?

2. If so, is patient interested in continuing therapy?

If patient is interested in continuing and is stable enough to do so, restart the infusion after reactions abate at a slower rate. Document the specifics of the reaction for future reference.

- Follow up with the patient in the next few days to assess for efficacy of the infliximab infusion.
- Premedicate the patient prior to subsequent infusions. Common combinations include acetaminophen along with diphenhydramine, but also with H_1 and H_2 blockers that are available over the counter.

3. Does the patient present with delayed hypersensitivity?

- The patient will likely call 6–10 days following an infusion with complaints of malaise, fever, diffuse arthralgias, and myalgias.
- If symptoms are mild (patient is ambulatory but uncomfortable), give acetaminophen prn.

- If symptoms are moderate, then give steroids 20 mg–40 mg per day until symptoms abate (usually 3–4 days) then taper rapidly.
- If symptoms are severe, that is, patient is unable to walk without assistance, consider hospitalization for IV fluids and steroids.

4. Are other medications needed for re-treatment with infliximab?

- If considering re-treatment with infliximab, pre-treatment with steroids, histamine blockers, and acetaminophen imperative.

III. TESTS TO ORDER

- Consider ordering infliximab levels and levels of antibodies to infliximab
- If no infliximab is present but there are antibodies greater than 8 μg/mL, then patient may not be a good candidate for re-treatment

CHAPTER 14

Complementary and Alternative Medicine

The use of complementary and alternative medicine (CAM) as well as visits to alternative practitioners continues to increase dramatically in the United States. Those involved with care of patients with IBD should be aware of common CAM approaches and knowledgeable about what information exists regarding safety and efficacy as well as to counsel patients appropriately.

Unfortunately, most of these approaches rely primarily on anecdotal reports spread through word of mouth or internet chat boards. Reliance on anecdotal evidence causes potentially very useful compounds such as probiotics to be mixed in with other reports that promote the benefits of ingesting foods as unlikely as gummy bears and coconut cookies as treatments for IBD.

Table 14.1. Partial list of alternative therapeutics in IBD

Oral Therapies
  Herbal supplements:
    Aloe vera
    Bach flower remedies
    Boswellia serrata
    Calendula
    Cat's claw
    Chamomile
    Ginseng
    Green tea
    Slippery elm
    Soy-derived isoflavones
  Vitamin supplements:

Alternative Medical Systems
  Ayurveda
  Homeopathy
  Naturopathy
  Traditional Chinese medicine

Probiotics/Prebiotics
  E. coli Nissle 1917
  Saccharomyces boulardii
  VSL#3
  PB8
  Homeostatic soil organisms/primal defense

Diet
  Low carbohydrate diet
  Rice-water diet
Specific Carbohydrate Diet

Physical Manipulation/Exercise
  Acupressure
  Acupuncture
  Aerobic exercise
  Chiropractic/osteopathy
  Feldenkrais
  Massage therapy
  Reiki
  Therapeutic touch

Mind–Body Interventions
  Distant healing
  Meditation
  Prayer
  Relaxation techniques

I. CONDITIONS TO CONSIDER

- Chronic disease
- Inflammatory bowel disease
- Significant or severe adverse events related to a conventional medication

II. QUESTIONS TO ASK

1. What is CAM?

- CAM is a broadly inclusive term referring to widely disparate therapies outside conventional biopsychosocial medicine:
  - herbal therapy
  - prayer healing
  - dance therapy
  - visualization
  - homeopathy

2. What do conventional practitioners think of all this?

- Defined in an early survey as "medical interventions not taught widely at U.S. medical schools or generally available at U.S. hospitals," CAM therapies are being adopted increasingly by the mainstream.

- The borders between some CAM and conventional medications are becoming blurred.

3. How prevalent is CAM use?

- Two identical surveys in 1991 and 1997 of the general population suggest an increase in CAM use in recent years.
  - Use of at least one of 16 different CAM therapies in the previous year had increased from 31% in 1990 to 41.6% in 1997.
  - Visits to alternative medicine practitioners increased as well from 36.3% to 46.3% in 1997.
  - The IBD population likely reflects this trend.

4. Do these figures differ from country to country?

- Surveys of CAM use vary widely depending in part on how CAM is defined as well as where the study is done.
- Surveys in different countries have estimated CAM use among people with IBD:
  - 31% (Cork, Ireland)
  - 47% (Berne, Switzerland)
  - 57% (Winnipeg, Canada)
  - 69% (Los Angeles, California).
  - CAM is used by a large percentage of people in the United States.

5. Who among IBD patients uses CAM therapies or visits CAM practitioners?

- Individuals are not easily profiled. Some studies have suggested that:
  - Women are more likely than men to use CAM.
  - Older individuals tend to use prayer, diet, and exercise as a therapeutic intervention more than younger individuals.
  - People who have had the disease for some time use CAM more frequently than those recently diagnosed.
  - Higher educational status also correlated with CAM use.

6. How reliable are these findings?

- Few of these findings have been identified consistently across studies.
- The characteristics of individuals more likely to use CAM are likely less applicable since the internet, which has become widely accessible, allows easy access to information and sources that direct people toward alternative approaches to their disease.

7. What motivates IBD patients to turn to CAM?

- The motivations for using these therapies are generally straightforward:
  - A powerful factor is the desire to be more in control of their lives in confronting a disease

that gives them a sense of lack of control versus a conventional medical approach.

- Some describe conventional medicine makes them passive participants in their own care.
- IBD patients consider CAM a genuinely complementary approach.
- Patients act from a willingness or eagerness to do whatever seems reasonable to them to improve their condition and maintain their health.
- Lack of effectiveness of conventional medications is a strong motivation for some.
- Most surveys do not find that disease activity correlates with the decision to use CAM.
  - IBD patients turning to CAM are not just the subgroup of people who fail to improve with conventional therapies or who have difficulty tolerating them.
  - Most individuals do not use CAM because of dissatisfaction with or rejection of conventional medication.

8. What types of CAM therapies do IBD patients use?

- Diet
- Exercise
- Mind healing (meditation, prayer, relaxation techniques, biofeedback)

- Physical manipulation (acupuncture, massage, acupressure, chiropractic, massage)
- Oral therapy (vitamins, herbals, probiotics, homeopathy)

9. What are the most commonly used therapies?

- Oral medications (including herbal remedies, which were 45% in one survey)
- Homeopathy
  - More popular abroad than in North America
    52% (Switzerland)
    16% (Canada)
  - Chiropractic (41%)
  - Massage therapy (23%)
  - Prayer (17%)
  - Relaxation techniques (17%)

10. What are the most popular herbal supplements?

- Aloe vera. An oral medication; often tried because of some evidence suggestive of improved healing, particularly in skin wounds.
  - A recent controlled trial of aloe vera (100 mL of aloe gel taken twice daily for 4 weeks) in 44 UC patients demonstrated a statistically significant benefit: in remission (30% vs. 7% in the placebo group), and in response (remission and improvement, 47% vs. 14%).

- A larger unpublished study of aloe vera in CD has been reported to have been negative.
- Other herbal supplements
  - cat's claw (*Uncaria tomentosa*)
  - *Boswellia serrata*
  - slippery elm
  - ginseng
  - green tea
  - soy-derived isoflavones
- Some animal data support the theoretical use of some of these compounds; human studies have not been performed.

11. What are a few of the diets IBD patients are following?

- The Specific Carbohydrate Diet (Gottschalk diet)
- Low carbohydrate diets
- Rice-water diets
- These approaches have not been adequately studied to cite reliable supporting data outside anecdotal reports.
  - For example, in IBD chat rooms and in other anecdotal reports, the most widely tried diet – the Specific Carbohydrate Diet – difficult for many to follow; remains controversial with strong advocates as well as critics.

12. What are probiotics and prebiotics?

- Probiotics. Live organisms that confer a health benefit.
- Prebiotics. Food ingredients that provide selective stimulation of growth or activity of beneficial native bacteria (i.e., a food source that selectively enhances the growth of specific bacteria).
- The particular species and dose, as with any medicine, is critical:
  - Probiotics (usually strains of bifidobacteria or *Lactobacillus*) sold as supplements in health food stores contain 10^9–10^{10} (1–10 billion) organisms per dose. Although seemingly a large amount, 1 gram of stool contains 10^{12} (1 trillion) bacteria.
- Supportive data
  - A broader scientific body of literature provides significant supporting rationale.
  - A number of placebo-controlled trials show supportive data for certain strains or blends including *E. coli* Nissle 1917 and VSL#3 (particularly in pouchitis with 17/20 remaining in remission at 9 months vs. 0/20 on placebo).
- Probiotics and prebiotics are now making a transition from the edge of CAM to mainstream medicine, particularly with regard to GI diseases.

13. Why are CAM therapies so attractive and what undesirable side effects can occur?

- They are "natural."
- They are presumed synonymous with "benign" or "virtually free of" side effects.
- Herbals or others have potentially both mild as well as serious side effects.
- A PDR exists that is a reference for use.

14. What other negatives show up in studies?

- Many IBD patients who use CAM do not report their use to their physicians, even when asked.
- In one survey, although many volunteered information to their primary care physician about using CAM, less than half told their gastroenterologist without being prompted.
- In another study, less than 10% of individuals who did not spontaneously report their CAM use responded accurately when asked by their physicians.

III. SOME CAVEATS

- CAM therapies hold the promise of benefit without adverse effects, but, as with conventional medications, these approaches should not be used cavalierly.

- Doses, duration of treatment, preparations, and potential interactions are factors that need to be evaluated and understood.
- There are few well-designed studies to guide their use.

PART FOUR

Special Populations

CHAPTER 15

The Post-Operative Patient

I. CONDITIONS TO CONSIDER

- Wound dehiscence/infection
- Abscess formation
- Anastomotic leaking
- Ischemia of anastomosis
- Small bowel obstruction
- Acute narcotic withdrawal
- Recurrent disease

II. QUESTIONS TO ASK

1. What are the patient's current symptoms?

- Sometimes over the phone you can tell whether this is a medical versus a surgical issue and the patient can be referred back to the surgeon.
- Any complaints about a wound or a stoma should be referred back to the surgeon.

2. When was the surgery?

- The differential will change when the surgery was 1 week versus about 2 months ago.

3. What procedure did the patient have done?

- A limited small bowel resection for Crohn's disease will have different complications compared with a patient who has had a total colectomy for ulcerative colitis.
- For UC, an ileal pouch anal anastomosis will be done in stages, and a retained rectum can bleed.

4. What medications is the patient taking?

- Patients taking a significant amount of narcotics could develop constipation, ileus, and small bowel obstruction. Acute withdrawal from narcotics can cause rebound pain or withdrawal-type symptoms.
- A patient with Crohn's who has not restarted maintenance medications may have an early recurrence if not all visible disease has been resected.
- Nonsteroidal medications may lead to anastomotic ulcers and bleeding, independent of any IBD.

5. What is the patient's current diet?

- A premature advancement or nonadherence to a low residue diet in the early postoperative period can lead to small bowel obstruction or diarrhea.

III. TESTS TO ORDER

- Physical exam. There is no substitute for seeing the patients if they are complaining of an infected wound, fever, obstructive symptoms, or abdominal pain/distension.
- CBC; electrolytes
- Amylase, lipase
- Consider wound, blood cultures
- X-ray. Plain film to rule out small bowel obstruction, free air
- CT scan to rule out abscess formation, free fluid, or pancreatitis.
- Endoscopy. Rarely needed in the early postoperative period; there will be edema secondary to the surgery itself that is not necessarily indicative of active disease.
- Helpful weeks to months post-op to rule out recurrent disease or ulcerations from other causes.

CHAPTER 16

The Pediatric IBD Patient

Children account for approximately 25% of all IBD cases. The median age at diagnosis is 12.5 years. CD is primarily seen in children of school age, outnumbering UC by approximately 3 to 1, but in the preschool group, UC is as frequent as CD. Although the clinical manifestations of IBD may be very similar among children and adults, key features of pediatric onset disease distinguish this population as unique:

I. CONDITIONS TO CONSIDER

- Growth failure
- Pubertal delay
- Proximal small bowel involvement
- Medication adherence
- Complex communication matrix
- Fear of procedures

- Depression and anxiety
- School absenteeism
- Family history
- Colon cancer risk
- Lack of indicated therapies

II. QUESTIONS TO ASK

1. Does the child have growth failure?

- At least 1/3 of children with CD yet only 1/10 children with UC present with growth failure. The presence of growth failure must increase the suspicion for CD involving the small bowel even despite what is considered an established diagnosis of UC.
- Growth failure can occur prior to the onset of any GI symptoms.
- The most common cause of growth failure is malnutrition, which is primarily a result of inadequate caloric intake.
- Other causes of malnutrition include increased intestinal losses, malabsorption, and increased energy requirements.
- Weight loss typically precedes linear growth failure.
- Pubertal delay is another manifestation of malnutrition and often accompanies linear growth delay.

- Active disease can contribute to ongoing growth failure.
- Corticosteroids can have a significant effect on growth velocity, and steroid dependency remains an unacceptable therapeutic end point for pediatric patients.
- Genetic and endocrine factors can certainly impact on growth and must be considered in the differential diagnosis of growth failure.

2. Are children adhering to their medications?

- Illness- and patient-related, family- and physician-related factors influence treatment adherence.
- The stage and course of the illness will impact treatment adherence.
- The psychological state of the child will impact on the adherence to treatment; positive self-esteem is an important predictor of adherence.
- The quality of family functioning will affect the adherence to therapies, and family disruption must be monitored.
- The importance of articulating a clear treatment plan cannot be stressed strongly enough when talking about ways of maximizing patient and family adherence.
- Physicians need to appreciate that socioeconomic classes and ethnicity may influence

beliefs and impact adherence to medical management.

- Peer support groups can enhance adherence by the exchange of medical information.
- Teens may acquire negotiation tools that differ from those of a younger age group; maintaining autonomy is important for adherence.
- Decreasing pill count and simplifying the timing of pill taking can increase medication compliance.

3. What is the psychosocial impact of IBD on the child?

- Maximizing the quality of life is an important outcome in the treatment of IBD patients.
- Children with IBD strive to fit in and not to be differentiated from their peers.
- It is uncommon for children with IBD to disclose their illness to children unaffected by IBD or other chronic diseases.
- School absenteeism, secondary to illness and hospitalizations, can impact on school performance and peer relationships.
- The esthetic and emotional side effects of certain medications – corticosteroids in particular – can significantly affect the psychosocial functioning of children.
- Depression and anxiety are not uncommon in children with IBD.

- Support groups and national camp programs may play a very important role in helping children and their families cope with disease and improve psychosocial functioning.

4. Is the natural history of IBD in children different than in adults?

- Disease onset before the age of 15 and disease duration are known risk factors for the development of colon cancer in UC.
- Chemopreventative measures with 5-ASA therapies and folic acid should be considered early in the course of disease.
- Screening colonoscopy after the age of 8 for extensive colitis and after 10 for left-sided colitis needs to be employed in children.
- Children with primary sclerosing cholangitis and colitis need to start their screening regimen at the time of diagnosis.
- CD onset before the age of 20 has been shown to be associated with a more aggressive disease course with patients undergoing more surgeries caused by medically refractory disease.
- Immunomodulators may be considered early in children presenting with extensive disease, steroid dependency, and growth failure.

5. Are the therapies used in children different from those used in adults?

- The therapeutic approach to children is essentially the same as that of adults with IBD.
- Both induction and maintenance therapies are used in children.
- The only therapies currently approved for use in children with IBD are corticosteroids and sulfasalazine.
- Mesalamine-based therapies remain first-line in patients with mild to moderate IBD.
- Nutritional supplementation is an important part of the treatment of a child, especially in the face of growth failure.
- Corticosteroids, although frequently used, can have significant impact on growth and thus only short-term courses are tolerated. There is no role for low-dose corticosteroids for the maintenance of disease remission.
- Immunomodulators, such as 6-MP/AZA and methotrexate (MTX), are very effective therapies employed for the maintenance of a steroid-free remission.
- Infliximab, although not approved for children, is frequently being used and the efficacy of this drug appears similar to that seen in adults (65% response rate). The safety profile similarly parallels that of adults with most pediatric patients tolerating this therapy.

- Infectious complications need to be monitored in all immunosuppressed patients whose treatments include corticosteroids.
- All immunosuppressed patients should receive annual protective shots against flu.
- Children on immunomodulators should not receive live vaccines.
- The surgical approaches to children with both CD and UC are similar to those in adults.

III. TESTS TO ORDER

In addition to the common endoscopic, radiologic, and laboratory tests that are ordered for all IBD patients, there are certain tests that may help to optimize the management of pediatric patients with IBD.

- Calorie count and nutritional consult to ensure adequate caloric intake to prevent growth failure
- Albumin, prealbumin, iron panel, and vitamin D levels can provide a very good baseline assessment of nutritional status and degree of malabsorption.
- Consider bone age in any child who presents with growth failure; bone age can provide information on catch-up growth potential when compared to chronological age.

- Bone density scan may not be very accurate in children if not compared with the appropriate age- and sex-matched population.
- WBC scan may be a noninvasive way of evaluating the presence of small bowel inflammation.
- CT scans should be used only when necessary in children given the cumulative radiation exposure risk over their lifetimes.
- Serum anti-*Saccharomyces cerevisiae* (ASCA) and antineutrophil antibodies (pANCA) may be helpful noninvasive tests in differentiating CD from UC in patients presenting with indeterminate colitis.
- Fecal calprotectin may be a helpful noninvasive test in predicting response to treatment and relapse in patients with IBD.
- Psychosocial evaluations for the patients and their families can be an important part of the overall management of patients with IBD.

CHAPTER 17

The Pregnant Patient

The highest age-adjusted incidence rates of IBD overlap the peak reproductive years. New medications are allowing patients to be healthier and disease-free for longer intervals, which may prompt a desire for conception. A pregnant IBD patient should be carefully monitored by both her gastroenterologist and her obstetrician for signs of active disease and fetal complications.

I. CONDITIONS TO CONSIDER

■ Fertility

- Women with UC and CD have similar and slightly lower rates of fertility, respectively, compared to the general population.

- Surgical intervention, such as a procto-colectomy with ileoanal pouch, can decrease fertility.

■ Disease Activity
- IBD activity is the strongest predictor of pregnancy outcome.
- Active IBD during conception can lead to higher rates of spontaneous abortion.
- Active IBD during the pregnancy can lead to higher rates of prematurity, small for gestational age (SGA) and low birth weight (LBW) infants. Patients have a 1/3 chance of flaring during pregnancy, similar to the general population, and should ideally be in remission prior to attempting conception.

■ Pregnancy Outcome
- Women with IBD have higher rates of premature birth.
- Women with active IBD at conception have higher rates of spontaneous abortion.

■ Fetal Outcome
- The majority of infants are normal and healthy.
- There is an increased risk of LBW and SGA infants.

- Congenital malformations do not appear to be higher, though the data are mixed.

II. COMMONLY ASKED QUESTIONS

1. What medications are safe to use during pregnancy?

- Methotrexate, thalidomide, and diphenoxylate are contraindicated in pregnancy.
- Metronidazole and ciprofloxacin are relative contraindications. Brief courses of metronidazole for 7–10 days may be used in the second and third trimesters. For IBD purposes, given their limited efficacy, these medications are not advised. Breast-feeding is not recommended.
- Mesalamine agents are safe in pregnancy and breast-feeding. If sulfasalazine is used, folic acid 2 mg daily should be given. Sulfasalazine is not known to cause kernicterus in the breast-fed infant.
- Prednisone is considered safe during pregnancy and can be used for flares. There is a risk of gestational diabetes and a theoretical risk of adrenal insufficiency in the infant. Breast-feeding is allowed.
- AZA and 6-MP are controversial. The majority of data in IBD supports their safety in pregnancy. The risks to the mother of flaring

should be balanced against the theoretical risk to the fetus.

- If the mother has a difficult disease, she can be managed on 6-MP/AZA throughout her pregnancy.
- Breast-feeding is relatively contraindicated due to the risk of immunosuppression and myelotoxicity. This should be individualized and discussed with the patient's specialist.

- Cyclosporine is safer than colectomy in the gravid UC patient with severe, steroid refractory disease. Fortunately, the need for it is rare.
- The safety of infliximab is unknown in pregnancy and breast-feeding. Data in more than 126 women receiving infliximab near conception do not show an increase in adverse events. A small case series of intentional use throughout pregnancy also did not demonstrate any adverse events.

2. What is the effect of smoking?

- Smoking has been shown to increase relapse rates, and decrease response to medications for Crohn's disease.
- For the health of the fetus (and the mother), the mother should be encouraged to stop smoking.

3. Does the patient have to have a C-section?

- In general, an IBD patient can have a normal spontaneous vaginal delivery unless obstetric indications suggest a Cesarean section.
- A patient with active perianal disease should have a Cesarean section.
- A patient with an ileal pouch anal anastomosis can deliver vaginally without harming the pouch. However, many surgeons recommend Cesarean sections because anal sphincter function, critical in these patients, may be compromised by a vaginal delivery either immediately or in the future.

III. TESTS TO ORDER

- Physical Exam. The patient with an ileostomy may develop obstruction, herniation, or other complications and should be examined regularly for this.
- Perianal disease should be ruled out prior to delivery.
- Anemia should be monitored.
- Drop in WBC count and hemoglobin, abnormal liver function, and pancreatitis may occur in the patient on 6-MP/AZA. These labs should be monitored closely as indicated during pregnancy.

- The fetus should be monitored regularly for evidence of SGA or LBW infants.
- Endoscopy for IBD is not usually needed during pregnancy. If there are severe symptoms, and the role of IBD is unclear, an unsedated flexible sigmoidoscopy can be performed safely.

CHAPTER 18

The Elderly Patient

IBD is not as rare in the elderly as previously believed. Although the majority of patients are diagnosed before they are 30 years old, there is a second smaller peak in disease incidence between the ages of 60 and 80; up to 20% of patients with UC and CD are elderly at the time of onset of symptoms. Diagnostic difficulties in the elderly include the lack of universally adopted diagnostic criteria, the misconception that IBD rarely has its onset in old age, the increasing number of diagnostic considerations with advancing age, and the frequency of atypical symptoms and findings in older patients with IBD.

Elderly patients who already have an established diagnosis of IBD are managed in a similar fashion to their younger counterparts in terms of disease flares. In the elderly patient with new symptoms such as bloody diarrhea or abdominal pain that are suggestive of IBD, a careful history and consideration of other conditions and exacerbating factors, particularly medications, must be taken into account.

I. CONDITIONS TO CONSIDER

- Ischemic colitis
- Infection: *Salmonella, Shigella, Campylobacter, Yersinia, C. difficile, E. coli* O157:H7
- Diverticular disease
- Microscopic colitis
- Radiation enterocolitis
- Malignancy
- Medications: NSAIDs, gold compounds, ticlopidine, phosphate soda preparations

II. QUESTIONS TO ASK

1. Does the patient already have an established diagnosis of IBD?

2. What are some common potential disease precipitants in patients with IBD and increased disease activity ?

- Stopping or decreasing IBD medications
- Starting antibiotics
- *C. difficile* coinfection

3. How severe are the symptoms?

- Although the elderly often respond to medical therapy as well as younger patients, the presence of comorbid conditions such as coronary artery disease, hypertension, peripheral vascular disease, and diabetes may result in a higher morbidity and mortality. A lower threshold for hospitalization may therefore be appropriate.

- Atypical symptoms are more common in the elderly: A change in mental status as a result of diarrhea and dehydration may be the presenting symptom in an older patient with peripheral vascular disease and hypertension.

- Concomitant *C. difficile* infection may manifest as an ileus and leukocytosis rather than diarrhea.

4. Is the patient taking any NSAIDs or aspirin?

- A higher prevalence of arthritis and coronary artery disease occurs in the elderly population. Elderly patients are therefore more likely to be taking NSAIDs and/or aspirin that may precipitate a flare.

- Remember to ask patients about over-the-counter NSAIDs in addition to prescription medications.

5. What medications are appropriate for the elderly IBD patient?

- Aminosalicylates are well tolerated.
- Azathioprine and 6-MP are also generally well tolerated, although given the slow onset of action, they are less beneficial in the acute setting.
- As with younger patients, there is often synergy between oral and topical (suppositories and enemas) medications.
- There is no reported difference in the efficacy or safety of infliximab in the elderly.
- Corticosteroids have a higher risk of complications in the elderly and must therefore be used judiciously. Side effects include osteoporosis, cataracts, glaucoma, diabetes, psychosis, depression, infections, electrolyte abnormalities, congestive heart failure, and hypertension.

6. What negative surgical outcomes are possible?

- Predictors of adverse postoperative outcome include preexisting health status, comorbid illnesses, severity of the acute attack, and the need for emergency surgery.
- Ileal pouch anal anastomosis may result in more erectile dysfunction and fecal incontinence in the elderly patient.

- The elderly patient will face more cardiac and respiratory complications and a longer mean postoperative hospital stay.
- No significant difference in frequency of anastomotic leaks in the elderly.

III. TESTS TO ORDER

- If the diagnosis is uncertain, colonoscopy with biopsy will often help to distinguish Crohn's disease and ulcerative colitis from other conditions (diverticular disease, ischemia, and so forth). Ischemia or infection may look like colitis at the time of colonoscopy, but the pathology should reveal characteristic differences.
- A CBC may reveal severe anemia indicative of active disease in a patient with a paucity of GI symptoms or atypical symptoms.
- Always consider *C. difficile* in a patient with worsening symptoms, even in the absence of recent antibiotic use.
- Vital signs and overall appearance in the elderly patient are as important as the abdominal exam and may indicate increased disease activity. Orthostasis and poor skin turgor may suggest dehydration, temporal wasting may be a sign of recent weight loss, altered mental status may be a sign of sepsis or shock.

PART FIVE

Special Considerations

CHAPTER 19

Colorectal Cancer in Inflammatory Bowel Disease

Patients newly diagnosed with IBD are faced with a bewildering array of emotional and physical problems; learning that this disease may also cause bowel cancer invariably brings anxiety and fear. These feelings should be addressed by their healthcare providers and may be ameliorated by helping patients understand their individual risks, describing the relative rarity of this complication, and engaging patients in effective prevention strategies.

I. CONDITIONS TO CONSIDER

- Chronic IBD
- Ulcerative colitis
- Crohn's disease of the bowel
- Precancerous dysplasia

II. QUESTIONS TO ASK

1. How prevalent is colorectal cancer?

- Although this is a rare complication of IBD, the morbidity and mortality associated with this complication have been well described, and prevention strategies have been developed.
- It is believed that the overall prevalence of CRC in UC is approximately 3.6%.

2. Who is most at risk for colorectal cancer?

- Patients with chronic inflammatory bowel disease have an increased risk for colorectal cancer (CRC).
- The majority of studies and published evidence regarding CRC in IBD is in UC, although the association in patients with CD of the colon has been increasingly reported and is now accepted as well.
- The risk increases as the duration of disease increases from approximately 2% after 10 years of disease to approximately 20% by 30 years of disease.

3. What are the known risk factors for dysplasia and CRC?

- In chronic UC (and probably Crohn's colitis), risk factors include those that are immutable:
  - Longer duration of disease
  - Greater extent of disease

Table 19.1. **Risks for dysplasia and cancer in chronic IBD**

Longer Duration of Disease
Greater Extent of Disease
Family History of Colorectal Cancer
Primary Sclerosing Cholangitis (PSC)
Younger Age of Diagnosis
Possibly Backwash Ileitis
Possibly Degree of Inflammation

- Family history of CRC (independent of a family history of IBD)
- Primary sclerosing cholangitis (PSC) and probably younger age of diagnosis
- Risk factors that are potentially modifiable, but remain incompletely proven include:
  - The degree of inflammation of the bowel
  - "Backwash ileitis," in which the small intestine adjacent to the ileocecal valve is exposed to inflammatory "backwash" through the ileocecal valve (Table 19.1).

4. Have any studies determined the cause of CRC?

- Colorectal cancer in IBD is thought to arise from precancerous dysplasia, which may progress from low-grade to high-grade before becoming invasive adenocarcinoma.

5. Can surveillance and surgery prevent CRC in IBD?

- Yes. Most CRC in IBD can be prevented if both patient and caregiver are educated

Table 19.2. **Guidelines for cancer prevention in IBD**

1. Ulcerative colitis or Crohn's colitis (without PSC) for > 8 years: surveillance colonoscopy with 3 or 4 biopsies every 10 cm, total approximately 33 biopsies. Repeat every 1–3 years depending on compounded risks. If the patient has PSC, see item 4.
2. If high-grade dysplasia is identified, confirm it by review of a second pathologist. If confirmed, recommend proctocolectomy. If low-grade dysplasia is identified, discuss proctocolectomy, refer for surgical consultation.
3. Encourage adherence to 5-ASA therapy ($\geq$ 1.2 g/d) for maintenance as well as for proposed chemopreventive properties.
4. If the patient has PSC, start surveillance at the time of diagnosis, and continue yearly. In addition, patients with PSC and UC should be on ursodeoxycholic acid 300 mg b.i.d.

---

about risks and follow published guidelines (Table 19.2).

- Prevention of CRC in IBD first requires risk stratification of the patient based on the compounded risk factors.
- A combination of surveillance colonoscopy and chemoprevention should be included.
- Recent work has shown that if not removed, low-grade dysplasia may progress to a higher grade or to cancer in at least 50% of cases over 5 years.

- It is important to have a frank discussion with the patient about these risks and emphasize that colorectal cancer is curable in its earliest stages.

6. Is the patient's age a factor in risk stratification?

- Yes, given the increased risk of sporadic CRC with advancing age.

7. Why should patients undergo scheduled colonoscopies?

- Surveillance colonoscopy is an effective prevention strategy:
  - Precancerous dysplasia is identified.
  - When CRC has already developed, it is found at an earlier stage.
  - Patients undergoing surveillance colonoscopy who develop CRC are more likely to have CRC at a lower stage, and have an associated improved survival than those who do not undergo surveillance.

8. How do patient and surgeon decide on a colectomy? on a proctocolectomy?

- Dysplasia occurs in the flat lining of the colon and is found by random biopsy. At the time of colectomy, there are often additional higher-grade lesions identified.
- Concurrent adenocarcinoma is found in the colons of patients who undergo colectomy for a finding of dysplasia between 19% (for

low-grade dysplasia) and 67% (for high-grade dysplasia).

- The diagnosis of high-grade dysplasia confirmed by more than one pathologist should always be treated by proctocolectomy.
- The diagnosis of low-grade dysplasia should prompt a surgical consultation and careful discussion of risks and benefits of proctocolectomy versus increased surveillance.

9. Are there effective prevention strategies using medication?

- A number of agents have been proposed to prevent the development of dysplasia and CRC in patients with long-standing colitis:
  - The gallstone dissolution agent ursodeoxycholic acid (URSO) is used to treat other biliary diseases.
  - URSO also has been shown to prevent dysplasia and cancer in patients with IBD and PSC at doses of 300 mg twice daily; this agent is now recommended independent of its therapeutic benefits for PSC alone.
  - It remains unknown whether URSO will be helpful in IBD patients without PSC.
    - 5-aminosalicylic acid (5-ASA), a mainstay of therapy for patients with UC, has an emerging role of chemoprevention of dysplasia and CRC in chronic UC.

- In several studies, use of 5-ASA at doses of 1.2 g/d or greater reduced the risk of cancer by between 72% and 80%. Although more work is needed, the efficacy and safety of 5-ASA for treatment of UC and maintenance of remission warrants use of this medication for potential chemoprevention.
- Educating patients about the possibility of chemoprevention likely will improve their adherence to therapy, and will have additional benefits in controlling their disease.

10. Where is research going and how is it getting there?

- Ongoing research is evaluating better ways to identify dysplasia using magnifying colonoscopes, special stains of the colonic mucosa, and fecal DNA markers.

III. TESTS TO ORDER

- Random biopsies
  - Unlike easy-to-identify polyps in people without IBD, dysplasia in IBD may occur in the flat lining of the colon, and requires these biopsies throughout the at-risk colon to identify it.
- Surveillance colonoscopy with random biopsies is performed after 8 years of disease and

repeated every 1–3 years with random biopsies looking for dysplasia, and additional biopsies of polyps, strictures, or masses.
- The exception is the patient with PSC, in whom surveillance colonoscopy should begin at the time of diagnosis and be repeated annually.

CHAPTER 20

Nutritional Issues

There are many theories about food and its relationship to inflammatory bowel disease. Few standards of care exist for the use of nutritional therapies in IBD, but we do know that excellent nutrition is essential to improve overall health in people with CD and UC.

I. CONDITIONS TO CONSIDER

- Weight loss
- Malnutrition
- Malabsorption of nutrients
- Lactose intolerance

II. QUESTIONS TO ASK

1. What is contributing to the malnutrition?

- Decreased nutrient intake may be secondary to loss of appetite and abdominal pain.

- Malabsorption/gastrointestinal losses can result in vitamin/mineral deficiencies and weight loss.
- Overly restricted diet.

2. How can the malnutrition be reversed?

- Consumption of adequate calories; most adult patients with IBD require 25–35 cal/kg of ideal body weight (IBW) and 1 g–1.5 g/kg IBW of protein/d.
- Frequent meals throughout the day to meet patient's nutritional requirements of calories, protein, vitamins, and minerals.
- Supplement with oral nutritional products if it is impossible for the patient to consume adequate nutrition with food alone. A concentrated formula may be indicated if a patient requires a large amount of supplemental calories (1.5 cal/cc).
- Vitamin/mineral supplementation. Patients with IBD are at risk for developing multiple vitamin and mineral deficiencies, most often secondary to inadequate intake of nutrients.
  - Folic acid. Sulfasalazine and methotrexate may alter folic acid absorption and metabolism; supplementation is recommended with 1 mg/d. Folic acid has also been found to protect patients against colon cancer.

- Vitamin D. Increased disease activity promotes deficiency and contributes to low bone mineral density (BMD) and osteoporosis; Vitamin D is the most common deficiency in CD.
- Vitamin B_{12}. Patients with ileal disease or resection of the ileum are at increased risk for deficiency; the terminal ileum is the site of absorption. Bacterial overgrowth may also increase the risk of vitamin B_{12} deficiency.
- Calcium. Corticosteroids can decrease the absorption of calcium; increased calcium in the diet and/or supplementation is necessary. Calcium is important for maintaining strong bones.
- Zinc. Severe diarrhea, enteric fistulas, and moderate-to-severe disease activity can result in deficiency.
- Iron. Deficiency is frequently seen in IBD, it can be secondary to decreased intake, increased losses, and/or decreased absorption. Recommended supplementation for deficiency is 150 mg–200 mg of elemental iron/d.

3. Does the patient require an alternative form of nutrition support?

- Yes, if the patient is unable to consume adequate nutrition orally and weight loss or failure to gain weight is a problem.

- Enteral nutrition (po/nasograstric/gastrostomy) can be used as supplemental nutrition to oral diet or as the sole source of nutrition therapy when oral intake is very poor or disease activity is severe.

  Studies have shown that nutritional therapy using enteral products may result in disease remission rates quite similar to rates achieved when corticosteroids are used. However, compliance can become an issue with enteral nutrition as sole source nutrition.

- Total parenteral nutrition (TPN) can be utilized when the enteral route is unable to be used or when bowel rest is necessary. There have been little data exploring the therapeutic effect of TPN on IBD although, based on the studies that have been completed, TPN appears to have more of a benefit for patients with CD than UC.

4. Should people with IBD avoid dairy products?

- Lactose intolerance has not been proved to affect patients with IBD more than the American population in general. The prevalence of lactose intolerance is greater in patients with CD affecting the small bowel than in patients with Crohn's colitis or UC.

- Symptoms of lactose intolerance include diarrhea, nausea, vomiting, abdominal cramps, bloating, and early satiety, which are symptoms that may be present with IBD.

- If there is a question whether or not someone is lactose intolerant, it is recommended that dairy products be removed from the diet and the patient monitored for improvement in symptoms. If no change is seen, slowly add the dairy back into the diet.

5. When is a low residue diet recommended?

- It may be recommended for certain IBD patients and may only be temporary. A low residue diet is usually followed until the inflammation responds to medical treatment.
- Patients with strictures or areas of narrowing may benefit from following a long-term, low residue diet to minimize abdominal pain, decrease other symptoms, and prevent obstructions from occurring.
- Patients following a low residue diet should avoid foods high in fiber, especially raw fruits and vegetables, seeds, nuts, and popcorn.

6. What is the difference between omega-3 and omega-6 fatty acids?

- Eicosapentaenoic acid (EPA) and docosahexaenoic acid (DHA), both omega-3 fatty acids, are found in fish oil. Omega-3 fatty acids have been found to have antiinflammatory properties and may decrease disease activity and the rate of relapse in CD patients who are in remission.

- It is hypothesized that following a Mediterranean-style diet, including fish and olive oil, is beneficial for patients with IBD. Additional studies are needed to clarify dosage and duration of treatment.
- Omega-6 fatty acids (safflower oil, corn oil, walnuts) should be avoided in the diet because they have proinflammatory properties.

7. Do probiotics help people with IBD?

- The gut flora plays an important role in maintaining normal intestinal function; a disturbance of the flora is seen in IBD. Probiotics may improve the microbial balance in the intestine, but further studies are needed to answer questions related to the benefit of probiotics and the dosage, duration, and frequency of treatment.

8. In summary, what nutritional therapy recommendations should IBD patients follow?

- Consumption of adequate calories to maintain a healthy weight or promote weight gain if indicated.
- Supplemental calories should be utilized, orally or enterally, based on the patient's needs.
- TPN should be used only if the GI tract is unable to be employed in feeding.

- A daily multivitamin should be administered, along with additional supplemental vitamins and minerals as needed (based on chemistry levels, drug therapy, and clinical findings).
- Unnecessary restrictions in the diet should be avoided to ensure optimal nutritional intake.

III. TESTS TO ORDER

- CBC
- Serum albumin
- Serum electrolytes
- Folic acid, vitamin B_{12}
- Serum iron, total iron-binding capacity, ferritin
- Serum calcium, magnesium, phosphorus
- Alkaline phosphatase (surrogate marker for zinc deficiency)
- Bone age (if growth impaired)
- Vitamin D
- Hydrogen breath testing is another way to test for lactose intolerance
- Additional tests if growth failure or significant malnutrition is present: Vitamins A, E, prothrombin time, zinc

CHAPTER 21

Osteoporosis

Osteoporosis, thinning of the bones, is a concern among many women, especially those who are experiencing or have experienced menopause. Osteoporosis accounts for 1.5 million fractures that result in over $13 billion in medical costs in the United States annually. It is estimated that over 5 million U.S. citizens have osteoporosis, and over 21 million have a precursor condition called "osteopenia."

By using a few simple rules, we can identify IBD patients at risk for osteoporosis, use a noninvasive screening tool to test them, and then choose an agent to reduce the future risk of fracture. Remember, prevention of a complication is always easier than treating one!

I. CONDITIONS TO CONSIDER

- Osteoporosis increases one's susceptibility to developing fractures of the bones in the wrist, ribs, vertebral spine, and hips, often with minimal trauma.
- Possible explanations for osteoporosis in IBD patients include:
  - Corticosteroids like prednisone have been known for years to have powerful effects on bone metabolism. Studies show that decreased bone density and increased fracture risk may occur within a few months of starting steroids. Even low-dose prednisone (5 mg daily) usage has been associated with fracture risk.
  - Other drugs such as cyclosporine and methotrexate may reduce bone density slightly.
  - CD patients with small bowel involvement, or with a history of small bowel resections, may not properly absorb calcium and/or vitamin D.

II. QUESTIONS TO ASK

1. At present, what groups are at high risk for osteoporosis?

- Although postmenopausal Caucasian women are at highest risk for osteoporosis and osteopenia, these conditions are occurring with increasing frequency in both men and non-Caucasian women.

2. What are some risk factors IBD and CD patients face?

- Numerous studies show that IBD patients, especially CD patients, are at increased risk for osteoporosis and osteopenia. Some population-based estimates suggest that osteoporosis may occur in as many as 1 in 7 CD patients, and osteopenia may occur in as many as 45%. No single reason explains why IBD is a risk factor for osteoporosis.

- Many patients with IBD have a low body mass index (BMI), and this is an independent risk factor for osteoporosis.

- IBD itself, especially CD, may be a risk factor. Low bone densities have been noted in newly diagnosed patients, even before they have received corticosteroids. It is thought that perhaps elevated levels of circulating inflammatory cytokines have negative effects on bone formation and resorption.

- Cigarette smoking is a risk factor for osteoporosis, and many CD patients have a history of former or current smoking.

3. Are there predictors for risk that we can recognize?

- The most important risk factors for osteoporosis in the general population – older age, female gender, and low body mass index – are still the most important predictors of osteoporosis in the IBD population.

4. Does low BMI correlate exactly with fracture risk?

- Not necessarily correlate exactly with fracture risk, so it is important to determine if IBD patients have an increased risk of fracture. Most studies of fracture risk in IBD suggest that IBD patients are anywhere from 15% to 45% more likely than the general population to develop an osteoporotic fracture (hip, spine, wrist, or ribs). In most, but not all, studies, the fracture risk seems slightly higher in CD.

  It is interesting to note that smaller studies (i.e., a few hundred patients) could not demonstrate an increased fracture risk, whereas larger studies (i.e., a few thousand) could. Therefore, we can reassure our patients that although their fracture risk is increased, it may not be as high as previously thought.

5. If the risk of fracture is elevated (but not "sky-high") in IBD, how do we decide which patients should be tested for osteoporosis?

- Blanket screening of all IBD patients would probably result in unnecessary testing. The IBD patients most at risk for fracture are post-menopausal women, patients with low body mass index, and those receiving steroids.

6. What measures can be used to treat IBD-associated osteoporosis?

- Lifestyle modifications such as regular exercise and cessation of cigarette smoking should be encouraged.
- Strongly consider the use of IBD medications that allow steroid-dependent patients to wean successfully off steroids. Examples include azathioprine, 6-mercaptopurine, methotrexate, and infliximab.

7. Do at-risk IBD patients need any vitamins and minerals to supplement their diets?

- Elemental calcium intake should be at least 1,200 mg daily. For patients who don't get this in their diets, calcium carbonate or calcium citrate supplement should be recommended.
- Vitamin D intake should range from 400 IU to 800 IU daily – higher levels may be required in patients with malabsorption or vitamin D deficiency. (Such deficiency should be corrected prior to treatment with a bisphosphonate.)

8. Should at-risk IBD patients be given hormone therapy?

- Estrogen seems to be falling out of favor after one study showed that the risks (increase in cardiovascular events and breast cancers) outweigh the benefits of combined estrogen–progestin therapy.

- However, selective estrogen receptor modulators such as raloxifene (Evista) may increase bone density and reduce fracture risk, but not at the cost of more breast cancers.
- Nasal salmon calcitonin spray (Miacalcin) has also been shown to be effective for improvement in bone density and reduction of fracture in the lumbar spine, primarily in women who are more than 5 years postmenopausal.
- Recombinant parathyroid hormone, or teriparatide (Forteo), when administered subcutaneously on a daily basis, can improve bone density and reduce fracture risk significantly.

  However, because of the observation of osteosarcomas in laboratory rats following administration of this drug, the FDA suggests that its use be limited to patients for whom the potential benefits are considered to outweigh the potential risk (i.e., those with previous history of osteoporotic fracture, multiple risk factors, or who have failed or are intolerant of other treatments); it is contraindicated in children and adolescents.

9. Are other medications being studied or given to these patients?

- Bisphosphonates block bone resorption. Two oral bisphosphonates, alendronate (Fosamax) and risedronate (Actonel), can be administered on either a daily or a weekly basis. Both medications have been shown to increase vertebral and femoral neck bone density and reduce vertebral and hip fractures for both postmenopausal and glucocorticoid-induced osteoporosis. In addition, risedronate prevents bone loss in patients receiving corticosteroids. Gastrointestinal side effects, including esophagitis, may occasionally occur with either medication, necessitating other treatment alternatives.

- Pamidronate (Aredia), 60 mg intravenously every 3 to 6 months, has been used by some physicians to deliver bisphosphonates for those who cannot tolerate oral preparations. Another intravenous bisphosphonate, zoledronic acid (Zometa), is currently being studied. Neither of these agents is approved by the FDA for use in osteoporosis.

III. TEST TO ORDER

- Dual-energy X-ray absorptiometry (DEXA) scanning. Several gastroenterological societies recommend that DEXA be performed in IBD patients with one or more of the following risk factors: age 60 years or older, low BMI, heavy smoking history, postmenopause, steroid treatment for at least 3 months, recurrent courses of steroids, and a history of prior fractures.

The results of a DEXA scan are usually given as a T-score. The T-score indicates the standard deviation from mean peak bone mass in the general population. In other words, a score of –3.0 indicates that the patient's bone density is 3 standard deviations below the mean, while a score of 0 would indicate a density exactly at the mean. A patient is considered to have osteoporosis if the T-score in the lumbar spine or hip or wrist is below –2.5, and osteopenia is defined as a T-score between –1.0 and –2.5.

CHAPTER 22

The Nonadherent Patient

So, your patient is feeling great and asks you, "Do I really need to take so much medicine? After all, it has been a while (thankfully) since I have had a flare of my disease." Yes, it is very important to continue to take maintenance medications. Here is a partial list why:

I. CONDITIONS TO CONSIDER

- IBD is a chronic, incurable disease, just like diabetes. You wouldn't tell diabetics to stop taking their insulin just because they feel well.
- The inflammation in the digestive tract is present even if the patients feel well, and it will get the better of them if they let it.
- IBD medications help to slow down the inflammatory process and promote healing, which

ultimately leads to the decreased risk of potential complications (like surgery).

II. QUESTIONS TO ASK

1. What else can happen when patients stop their medications?

- Not taking medications can lead to more aggressive flare-ups that may require steroid therapy, hospitalization, or surgery. The long-term consequences of steroids are well known and include cataract formation, osteoporosis, and poor skin healing.

2. Have any studies evaluated the long-term risks of a patient discontinuing taking medications?

- Several studies have shown what even short-term discontinuation of medications can do, especially if patients have required long courses of steroids in the past.

- A study performed at the University of Chicago followed well patients for 2 years. The study showed that patients had a *fivefold* increased risk for a disease flare of UC when they took less than 80% of their prescribed medication over that time period. Patients who continued on their medications regularly were less likely to have to visit their doctors, less likely to have procedures, and ultimately saved money.

- There have been 2 studies to show that patients taking long-term azathioprine for their CD are at risk for a flare if they stop taking it, even when they have been well for close to 5 years.
- Another study done at the University of Chicago, along with 5 studies done at other institutions, has shown that taking certain medicines like Asacol may decrease the risk of developing cancer.

3. Why do patients stop taking their medications?

- Most physicians don't do a good job at explaining what medications do, and the importance of their continued use.
- Patients are sometimes too embarrassed to admit they don't know what their medication does, that it costs too much, or that they are not taking it.

4. Who is more likely to not take their medications?

- Those patients who do not have a good support system. This includes single people and young college students.
- Males seem to be particularly susceptible to this behavior.

5. How do we as physicians combat this problem?

- We involve others – friends or organizations such as the Crohn's and Colitis Foundation of America (CCFA) so that patients do not feel so alone.

6. How can doctors help patients help themselves improve medication-taking behavior?

- Make things easy for them. Here is a list of suggestions to make to your patients:
  - Tell them whether they can take their medicines twice a day or even once a day rather than 3 or 4 times a day.
  - They can put their pills in several places so that when it is time to take their medications, they have some available. Taking the pills "later" often leads to skipped doses.
  - Explain what they should do if they miss a dose. Do they double the next one or just forget about it? There can be consequences to missing too many doses that should be discussed with your patient.

III. OTHER STEPS TO TAKE

- Open dialogues between the patient, the physician, and the others of the healthcare team are the best way to address concerns so that complications can be avoided.
- Make sure you know every medication your patients are taking. You, the doctor, may not agree, but at least you can then monitor for unwanted or unexpected side effects that may occur because of another pill the patients are taking without your knowledge.

- Encourage patients to ask you questions! If they don't understand what a pill does or what they should expect from it, then it cannot help them and they are less likely to take it.
- If they are having trouble paying for the medication, give them generic formulations, and tell them about patient assistance programs.

Selected References

Farmer RG, Easley K, Rankin GB. Clinical patterns, natural history, and progression of ulcerative colitis. Dig Dis Sci 1993;**38**:1137–1146.

Fireman, Z, et al. Epidemiology of Crohn's disease in the Jewish population of central Israel, 1970–1980. Am J Gastroenterol 1989;**84**(3):255–258.

Gionchetti P, Rizzello F, Venturi A, Brigidi P, Matteuzzi D, Bazzocchi G, Poggioli G, Miglioli M, Campieri M. Oral bacteriotherapy as maintenance treatment in patients with chronic pouchitis: a double-blind, placebo-controlled trial. Gastroenterology 2000;**119**:305–309.

Hendriksen C, Kreiner S, Binder V. Long-term prognosis in ulcerative colitis-based on results from a regional patient group from the county of Copenhagen. Gut 1985;**26**:158–163.

Hilsden RJ, Verhoef MJ, Best A, Pocobelli G. Complementary and alternative medicine use by

Canadian patients with inflammatory bowel disease: results from a national survey. Am J Gastroenterol 2003;**98**:1563–1568.

Jewell DP. Ulcerative colitis. In: Feldman M, Scharschmidt BF, Slesisenger MH, eds. Gastrointestinal and Liver Disease, vol 2, 6th ed. Philadelphia, PA: WB Saunders Co;1998:1735–1761.

Kessler RC, Davis RB, Foster DF, Van Rompay MI, Walters EE, Wilkey SA, Kaptchuk TJ, Eisenberg DM. Long-term trends in the use of complementary and alternative medical therapies in the United States. Ann Intern Med 2001;**135**:262–268.

Kornbluth A, Sachar DB. Ulcerative colitis practice guidelines in adults. American College of Gastroenterology. Practice Parameters Committee. Am J Gastroenterol 1997;**92**:204–211.

Kurata, JH, et al., Crohn's disease among ethnic groups in a large health maintenance organization. Gastroenterology 1992;**102**(6):1940–1948.

Langmead L, Feakins RM, Goldthorpe S, Holt H, Tsironi E, De Silva A, Jewell DP, Rampton DS. Randomized, double-blind, placebo-controlled trial of oral aloe vera gel for active ulcerative colitis. Aliment Pharmacol Ther 2004;**19**:739–747.

Loftus, EV Jr. Clinical epidemiology of inflammatory bowel disease: incidence, prevalence, and environmental influences. Gastroenterology 2004;**126**(6):504–517.

Quattropani C, Ausfeld B, Straumann A, Heer P, Seibold F. Complementary alternative medicine in patients with inflammatory bowel disease: use and attitudes. Scand J Gastroenterol 2003;**38**:277–282.

Rao SSC, Holdsworth CD, Read. Symptoms and stool patterns in patients with ulcerative colitis. Gut 1988;**29**:342–345.

Rawsthorne P, Shanahan F, Cronin NC, Anton PA, Lofberg R, Bohman L, Bernstein CN. An international survey of the use and attitudes regarding alternative medicine by patients with inflammatory bowel disease. Am J Gastroenterol 1999 May;**94**(5):1298–1303.

Rembacken BJ, Snelling AM, Hawkey PM, Chalmers DM, Axon AT. Non-pathogenic Escherichia coli versus mesalazine for the treatment of ulcerative colitis: a randomised trial. Lancet 1999;**354**:635–639.

Index